ICD-10 CM, AN ELEMENTARY APPROACH:
A GUIDE BY
XAIVER RAUF NEWMAN AHI, CEHRS, CORST

Introduction:

For many years, we've heard the rumors that this is the year that we change from ICD-9-CM to ICD-10-CM. Now, the word is factual, it's no rumor. We will be changing from using ICD-9-CM to ICD-10-CM not in 2011, not in 2012 but in 2013. ICD-10-CM will become effective as of October 1, 2013. This can be verified by going to the CMS. Their ICD-10 website located at https://www.cms.gov/ICD10/

The intent of this guide is NOT to scare you. This guide does NOT provide any information regarding ICD-10-PCS. I will leave ICD-10-PCS to the appropriate coding associations/organizations. The intent of this guide is to help you and to calm your fears. I do wish to say the following: First and foremost, I am a coder. I am NOT one of the nation's experts on ICD-10. I've looked at ICD-10 for the past two years and I've seen how simple it is and how using ICD-10 won't be that difficult. I've looked at all of the ICD-10 information that has been available from the Centers for Disease Control, the World Health Organization, the Centers for Medicare and Medicaid Services, the American Medical Association, the American College of Emergency Physicians, and the American Health Information Management Association since 2008. I use my background as a Hospital Corpsman, Certified Electronic Health Records Specialist, a coding and billing instructor for several Allied Health Programs, and curriculum writer to drawn upon.

Since the word came that ICD-10-CM was going to take place, there are many companies that are offering ICD-10-CM training. Some are using scare tactics such as, "Did you know that if you don't take our ICD-10 training, your claims won't be paid?"

First, let me say that there will always rumors. There are also companies that are willing to separate you from your money. I am selling this guide, but I didn't create it with intentions of general gain. It is being provided to you to destroy any insecurities or apprehension of ICD-10 interpretation. If you wish to attend any training sessions that are offered, you have the freedom of choice to do so. My recommendation is to take your training from reliable organizations and associations such as the AAPC, PAHCS, MAB, POMAA, or ELI Research. Several years ago, a company I worked for was scared into sending our coders to specialized "Medicare" training because we were told that if we didn't have this training, our claims wouldn't be paid. The training turned out to be a high-pressure sales tactic to buy books they were selling like "snake oil" or "tonic" in the old west.

Currently, there are no State or Federal laws that mandate that a specific teaching company or organization train your coding staff. Nor are there any State or Federal law requirements that your coders have to be certified. I say this because I am asked questions about certification on an almost daily basis. I am not a lawyer and I never provide legal advice, however, I and many of my colleagues do research on State laws for many clients so that they do not violate laws when coding or billing for providers in a given state. I will say that certification is a personal preference or an employer preference. I may get a request from a billing company in Johnson City, New York and they were hired to code and bill for an emergency practice in Clarksville, Iowa. I will research all of the Iowa Statutes and Administrative codes to find those laws or statutes that are important to the biller and coders.

I look to see if a coder or biller is mandated to be certified or registered by the State in addition to claim submission timeframes, coding specifics for workers compensation or auto accidents, Medicaid requirements and emergency care laws if the provider renders emergency care. Again, certification is both a personal and employer preference, but this does not mean this won't change in the future. For example: Mary Jones completes her coding training at Lake-Sumter Community College in Orlando Florida. Florida Law does not require a coder to be certified, licensed or registered. Mary wants to be certified in coding, so she takes the coding exams offered by the American Academy of Professional Coders (AAPC). John Smith was in the same class with Mary, he too wishes to become certified in coding, instead of becoming certified by the AAPC, he takes the coding certification test offered by the Professional Association of Healthcare Coding Specialists (PAHCS). John and Mary visit the medical practice of Dr. Patel. Dr. Patel is looking for a coder and he prefers a coder who is certified with the AAPC. Across the complex, Dr. Seuss also needs a coder and he prefers a coder who is certified through PAHCS. In the same complex, Dr. Doolittle also needs a coder but he has no preference to require a coder to be certified. His preference is a coder with 5 years of coding experience. The local hospital is currently hiring coders, but they want a coder to be certified by the AAPC.

They see that John is certified by PAHCS, so they make a provisional change so that they can hire John as a coder in addition to Mary being hired. John will be required to become AAPC certified within six months of being hired. On a personal note, I was trained in coding by Sharon Morikone, who, to me is the country's expert on coding emergency medicine. She was very tough. She could make a hard core Marine drill sergeant cry with her demand for 100% perfection. To be considered for any coding position, she demanded the candidate to take a coding test, using HIPAA sanitized medical records of real patients. The candidate had to train under her personal supervision for at least 6 months. During the training, you had to be 100% correct with your coding. It was so hard; I saw AAPC certified nurse's quit after an hour of training. Once you went through her supervised additional training, you were allowed to code on a provisional basis for another six months. If you made no errors during this period, you were allowed to code without supervision, but she still reviewed your work on a constant basis. If you were called to her office, it was scarier than visiting the Wizard of Oz. I am tentatively certified in coding by the Professional Association of Healthcare Coding Specialists (PAHCS) and the Physician Office Managers Association of America (POMAA), but those certifications are based on personal preference. The doctors who hired me accepted these coding certifications.

As a coder, I've looked at ICD-10-CM, and from a trained coders perspective, ICD-10-CM is not scary at all. I don't see anything mysterious. If you understand and know the process of diagnosis coding, you should have no problem with ICD-10-CM. Those that might have a problem are those who don't have any training and they were placed into the coding position within a doctor's practice. Many of these people now rely on the coding and billing forums to code for them. They go to the forum and they ask a question similar to the following: *"I forgot how to code this: A patient came in for a cranialrectalectomy, what diagnosis codes can I use to get this paid or what is the diagnosis code for XXXX?"*

ICD-9-CM has the following coding conventions:

A. Conventions for the ICD-9-CM

The conventions for the ICD-9-CM are the general rules for use of the classification independent of the guidelines. These conventions are incorporated within the index and tabular of the ICD-9-CM as instructional notes. The conventions are as follows:

1. Format:

The ICD-9-CM uses an indented format for ease in reference

2. Abbreviations

a. Index Abbreviations

NEC "Not elsewhere classifiable"

This abbreviation in the index represents "other specified." When a specific code is not available for a condition the index directs the coder to the "other specified" code in the tabular.

b. Tabular Abbreviations NEC "Not

elsewhere classifiable"

This abbreviation in the tabular represents "other specified." When a specific code is not available for a condition the tabular includes an NEC entry under a code to identify the code as the "other specified" code.

(See Section I.A. 5.a. "Other" codes)

NOS "Not otherwise specified"

This abbreviation is the equivalent of unspecified.

(See Section I.A. 5.b., "Unspecified" codes)

3. Punctuation

[ ] Brackets are used in the tabular list to enclose synonyms, alternative wording or explanatory phrases. Brackets are used in the index to identify manifestation codes.

(See Section I.A. 6. "Etiology/manifestations ")

( ) Parentheses are used in both the index and tabular to enclose supplementary words which may be present or absent in the statement of a disease or procedure without affecting the code number to which it is assigned. The terms within the parentheses are
referred to as nonessential modifiers.

: Colons are used in the Tabular list after an incomplete term which needs one or more of the modifiers following the colon to make it assignable to a given category.

4. Includes and Excludes Notes and Inclusion terms

Includes: This note appears immediately under a three-digit code title to further define, or give examples of, the content of the category.

Excludes: An excludes note under a code indicates that the terms excluded from the code are to be coded elsewhere. In some cases the codes for the excluded terms should not be used in conjunction with the code from which it is excluded. An example of this is a congenital condition excluded from an acquired form of the same condition. The congenital and acquired codes should not be used together. In other cases, the excluded terms may be used together with an excluded code. An example of this is when fractures of different bones are coded to different codes. Both codes may be used together if both types of fractures are present.

Inclusion terms: List of terms are included under certain four and five digit codes. These terms are the conditions for which that code number is to be used. The terms may be synonyms of the code title, or, in the case of "other specified" codes, the terms are a list of the various conditions assigned to that code. The inclusion terms are not necessarily exhaustive. Additional terms found only in the index may also be assigned to a code.

5. Other and Unspecified codes

a. "Other" codes

Codes titled "other" or "other specified" (usually a code with a 4th digit 8 or fifth-digit 9 for diagnosis codes) are for use when the information in the medical record provides detail for which a specific code does not exist. Index entries with NEC in the line designate "other" codes in the tabular. These index entries represent specific disease entities for which no specific code exists so the term is included within an "other" code.

b. "Unspecified" codes

Codes (usually a code with a 4th digit 9 or 5th digit 0 for diagnosis codes) titled "unspecified" are for use when the information in the medical record is insufficient to assign a more specific code.

6. Etiology/manifestation convention ("code first", "use additional code" and "in diseases classified elsewhere" notes)

Certain conditions have both an underlying etiology and multiple body system manifestations due to the underlying etiology. For such conditions the ICD-9-CM has a coding convention that requires the underlying condition be sequenced first followed by the manifestation. Wherever such a combination exists there is a "use additional code" note at the etiology code, and a "code first" note at the manifestation code. These instructional notes indicate the proper sequencing order of the codes, etiology followed by manifestation.

In most cases the manifestation codes will have in the code title, "in diseases classified elsewhere." Codes with this title are a component of the etiology/ manifestation convention. The code title indicates that it is a manifestation code. "In diseases classified elsewhere" codes are never permitted to be used as first listed or principal diagnosis codes. They must be used in conjunction with an underlying condition code and they must be listed following the underlying condition.

There are manifestation codes that do not have "in diseases classified elsewhere" in the title. For such codes a "use additional code" note will still be present and the rules for sequencing apply.

In addition to the notes in the tabular, these conditions also have a specific index entry structure. In the index both conditions are listed together with the etiology code first followed by the manifestation codes in brackets. The code in brackets is always to be sequenced second.

The most commonly used etiology/manifestation combinations are the codes for Diabetes mellitus, category 250. For each code under category 250 there is a use additional code note for the manifestation that is specific for that particular diabetic manifestation. Should a patient have more than one manifestation of diabetes more than one code from category 250 may be used with as many manifestation codes as are needed to fully describe the patient's complete diabetic condition? The category 250 diabetes codes should be sequenced first, followed by the manifestation codes.

"Code first" and "Use additional code" notes are also used as sequencing rules in the classification for certain codes that are not part of an etiology/ manifestation combination.

See Section I.B.9. "Multiple coding for a single condition".

7. "And"

The word "and" should be interpreted to mean either "and" or "or" when it appears in a title.

8. "With"

The word "with" in the alphabetic index is sequenced immediately following the main term, not in alphabetical order.

9. "See" and "See Also"

The "see" instruction following a main term in the index indicates that another term should be referenced. It is necessary to go to the main term referenced with the "see" note to locate the correct code.

A "see also" instruction following a main term in the index instructs that there is another main term that may also be referenced that may provide additional index entries that may be useful. It is not necessary to follow the "see also" note when the original main term provides the necessary code.

ICD-10-CM Coding Conventions:

A. Conventions for the ICD-10-CM

The conventions for the ICD-10-CM are the general rules for use of the classification independent of the guidelines. These conventions are incorporated within the Index and Tabular of the ICD-10-CM as instructional notes.

The Alphabetic Index and Tabular List

The ICD-10-CM is divided into the Index, an alphabetical list of terms and their corresponding code, and the Tabular List, a chronological list of codes divided into chapters based on body system or condition. The Index is divided into two parts, the Index to Diseases and Injury, and the Index to External Causes of Injury. Within the Index of Diseases and Injury there is a Neoplasm Table and a Table of Drugs and Chemicals.

See Section I. C2. General guidelines
See Section I.C. 19. Adverse effects, poisoning, underdosing and toxic effects

Format and Structure:

The ICD-10-CM Tabular List contains categories, subcategories and codes. Characters for categories, subcategories and codes may be either a letter or a number. All categories are 3 characters. A three-character category that has no further subdivision is equivalent to a code. Subcategories are either 4 or 5 characters. Codes may be 4, 5, 6 or 7 characters. That is, each level of subdivision after a category is a subcategory. The final level of subdivision is a code. All codes in the Tabular List of the official version of the ICD-10-CM are in bold. Codes that have applicable 7th characters are still referred to as codes, not subcategories. A code that has an applicable 7th character is considered invalid without the 7th character.

The ICD-10-CM uses an indented format for ease in reference

Use of codes for reporting purposes

For reporting purposes only codes are permissible, not categories or subcategories, and any applicable 7th character is required.

Placeholder character

The ICD-10-CM utilizes a placeholder character "X". The "X" is used as a 5th character placeholder at certain 6 character codes to allow for future expansion. An example of this is at the poisoning, adverse effect and underdosing codes, categories T36-T50. Where a placeholder exists, the X must be used in order for the code to be considered a valid code.

7th Characters
Certain ICD-10-CM categories have applicable 7th characters. The applicable 7th character is required for all codes within the category, or as the notes in the Tabular List instruct. The 7th character must always be the 7th character in the data field. If a code that requires a 7th character is not 6 characters, a placeholder X must be used to fill in the empty characters.

Abbreviations
   a. Index abbreviations
NEC "Not elsewhere classifiable"
This abbreviation in the Index represents "other specified". When a specific code is not available for a condition, the Index directs the coder to the "other specified" code in the Tabular.

   b. Tabular abbreviations
NEC "Not elsewhere classifiable"
This abbreviation in the Tabular represents "other specified". When a specific code is not available for a condition the Tabular includes an NEC entry under a code to identify the code as the "other specified" code.

NOS "Not otherwise specified"
This abbreviation is the equivalent of unspecified.

Punctuation
   [ ] Brackets are used in the tabular list to enclose synonyms, alternative wording or explanatory phrases. Brackets are used in the Index to identify manifestation codes.

   ( ) Parentheses are used in both the Index and Tabular to enclose supplementary words that may be present or absent in the statement of a disease or procedure without affecting the code number to which it is assigned. The terms within the parentheses are referred to as nonessential modifiers: Colons are used in the Tabular List after an incomplete term which needs one or more of the modifiers following the colon to make it assignable to a given category.

Use of "and"

When the term "and" is used in a narrative statement it represents and/or.

Other and Unspecified codes

a. "Other" codes

Codes titled "other" or "other specified" are for use when the information in the medical record provides detail for which a specific code does not exist. Index entries with NEC in the line designate "other" codes in the Tabular. These Index entries represent specific disease entities for which no specific code exists so the term is included within an "other" code.

b. "Unspecified" codes

Codes (usually a code with a 4th digit 9 or 5th digit 0 for diagnosis codes) titled "unspecified" are for use when the information in the medical record is insufficient to assign a more specific code. For those categories for which an unspecified code is not provided, the "other specified" code may represent both other and unspecified.

Includes Notes

This note appears immediately under a three-digit code title to further define, or give examples of, the content of the category.

Inclusion terms

List of terms is included under some codes. These terms are the conditions for which that code is to be used. The terms may be synonyms of the code title, or, in the case of "other specified" codes, the terms are a list of the various conditions assigned to that code. The inclusion terms are not necessarily exhaustive. Additional terms found only in the Index may also be assigned to a code.

Excludes Notes

The ICD-10-CM has two types of excludes notes. Each type of note has a different definition for use but they are all similar in that they indicate that codes excluded from each other are independent of each other.

a. Excludes 1

A type 1 Excludes note is a pure excludes note. It means, "NOT CODED HERE!" An Excludes1 note indicates that the code excluded should never be used at the same time as the code above the Excludes1 note. An Excludes1 is used when two conditions cannot occur together, such as a congenital form versus an acquired form of the same condition.

b. Excludes2

A type 2 excludes note represents "Not included here". An excludes2 note indicates that the condition excluded is not part of the condition represented by the code, but a patient may have both conditions at the same time. When an Excludes2 note appears under a code, it is acceptable to use both the code and the excluded code together, when appropriate.

Etiology/manifestation convention ("code first", "use additional code" and "in diseases classified elsewhere" notes)

Certain conditions have both an underlying etiology and multiple body system manifestations due to the underlying etiology. For such conditions, the ICD-10-CM has a coding convention that requires the underlying condition be sequenced first followed by the manifestation. Wherever such a combination exists, there is a "use additional code" note at the etiology code, and a "code first" note at the manifestation code. These instructional notes indicate the proper sequencing order of the codes, etiology followed by manifestation.

In most cases the manifestation codes will have in the code title, "in diseases classified elsewhere." Codes with this title are a component of the etiology/ manifestation convention. The code title indicates that it is a manifestation code. "In diseases classified elsewhere" codes are never permitted to be used as first listed or principal diagnosis codes. They must be used in conjunction with an underlying condition code and they must be listed following the underlying condition. See category F02, Dementia in other diseases classified elsewhere, for an example of this convention.

There are manifestation codes that do not have "in diseases classified elsewhere" in the title. For such codes a "use additional code" note will still be present and the rules for sequencing apply.

In addition to the notes in the Tabular, these conditions also have a specific Index entry structure. In the Index both conditions are listed together with the etiology code first followed by the manifestation codes in brackets. The code in brackets is always to be sequenced second.

An example of the etiology/manifestation convention is dementia in Parkinson's disease. In the index, code G20 is listed first, followed by code F02.80 or F02.81 in brackets. Code G20 represents the underlying etiology, Parkinson's disease, and must be sequenced first, whereas codes F02.80 and F02.81 represent the manifestation of dementia in diseases classified elsewhere, with or without behavioral disturbance.

"Code first" and "Use additional code" notes are also used as sequencing rules in the classification for certain codes that are not part of an etiology/ manifestation combination. *See Section I.B. 7. Multiple coding for a single condition.*

"And"

The word "and" should be interpreted to mean either "and" or "or" when it appears in a title.

"With"

The word "with" in the Alphabetic Index is sequenced immediately following the main term, not in alphabetical order.

"See" and "See Also"

The "see" instruction following a main term in the Index indicates that another term should be referenced. It is necessary to go to the main term referenced with the "see" note to locate the correct code.

A "see also" instruction following a main term in the index instructs that there is another main term that may also be referenced that may provide additional index entries that may be useful. It is not necessary to follow the "see also" note when the original main term provides the necessary code.

"Code also note"

A "code also" note instructs that two codes may be required to fully describe a condition, but this note does not provide sequencing direction.

Default codes

A code listed next to a main term in the ICD-10-CM Index is referred to as a default code.

005.0 The default code represents that condition that is most commonly associated with the main term, or is the unspecified code for the condition. If a condition is documented in a medical

005.1 record (for example, appendicitis) without any additional information, such as acute or chronic, the default code should be assigned.

005.2 Syndromes

Follow the Alphabetic Index guidance when coding syndromes. In the absence of index guidance, assign codes for the documented manifestations of the syndrome.

As you can see, the guidelines for ICD-9-CM are not that different than those for ICD-10-CM.

If you look at the following, you can see the similarity between ICD-9-Cm and ICD-10-CM:

ICD-9-CM

005 Other food poisoning (bacterial)

Excludes: salmonella infections *(003.0-003.9) toxic effect of:*

food contaminants (989.7)
noxious foodstuffs (988.0-988.9)

Staphylococcal food poisoning
Staphylococcal toxemia specified as due to food Botulism food poisoning

Botulism NOS
Food poisoning due to Clostridium botulinum *Excludes:*
infant botulism (040.41)
wound botulism (040.42)

Food poisoning due to Clostridium perfringens [C. welchii]
Enteritis necroticans

ICD-10-CM

A05 Other bacterial foodborne intoxications, not elsewhere classified

> *Excludes:* Escherichia coli infection (A04.0-A04.4)
> listeriosis (A32.-)
> salmonella foodborne intoxication and infection (

A05.0 **Foodborne staphylococcal intoxication**

A05.1 **Botulism**

Classical foodborne intoxication due to Clostridium botulinum

A05.2 **Foodborne Clostridium perfringens [Clostridium welchii] intoxication**

Enteritis necroticans Pig-bel

A05.3 **Foodborne Vibrio parahaemolyticus intoxication**

A05.4 **Foodborne Bacillus cereus intoxication**

A05.8 **Other specified bacterial foodborne intoxications**

A05.9 **Bacterial foodborne intoxication, unspecified**

As you can see there isn't too much difference between how ICD-9-CM and ICD-10-CM looks. Code 005 series becomes A05 series. You can see that the coding conventions still take place with ICD-10-CM.

If you look at the introduction of each section of ICD-9-CM, they are similar to the instructions in

ICD-10-CM: **ICD-9-CM**

1. INFECTIOUS AND PARASITIC DISEASES (001-139.8)

Includes: diseases generally recognized as communicable or transmissible as well as a few diseases of unknown but possibly infectious origin

Excludes: acute respiratory infections *(460-466)*
  carrier or suspected carrier of infectious organism *(V02.0-V02.9)*
  certain localized infections
  influenza *(487.0-487.8, 488)*

Note: Categories for "late effects" of infectious and parasitic diseases are to be found at 137-139.

ICD-10-CM

Certain infectious and parasitic diseases (A00-B99)

Includes: diseases generally recognized as communicable or transmissible

Use additional code (U80-U89), if desired, to identify the antibiotic to which a bacterial agent is resistant.

Excludes: carrier or suspected carrier of infectious disease (Z22.-)
  certain localized infections - see body system-related chapters
  infectious and parasitic diseases complicating pregnancy, childbirth and the puerperium [except obstetrical tetanus and human immunodeficiency virus [HIV] disease] (O98.-)
  infectious and parasitic diseases specific to the perinatal period [except tetanus neonatorum, congenital syphilis, perinatal gonococcal infection and perinatal human immunodeficiency virus [HIV] disease] (P35-P39)
  influenza and other acute respiratory infections (J00-J22)

Index Comparisons:

When we look at the Index of ICD-9-CM and ICD-10-CM, we can, again, see similarities: **ICD-9-CM**

AAT (alpha-1 antitrypsin) deficiency 273.4

AAV (disease) (illness) (infection)--*see* **Human immunodeficiency virus** (disease) (illness) (infection)

Abactio--*see* **Abortion, induced**

Abactus venter--*see* **Abortion, induced**

Abarognosis 781.9 View Subentries

Abderhalden-Kaufmann-Lignac syndrome (cystinosis) 270.0

Abdomen, abdominal--*see also* condition   View Subentries

Abdominalgia 789.0 View Subentries

Abduction contracture, hip or other joint--*see* **Contraction, joint**

Abercrombie's syndrome (amyloid degeneration) 277.39

ICD-10-CM

Aarskog's syndrome Q87.1
Abandonment - see Maltreatment, abandonment
Abasia (-astasia) (hysterical) F44.4
Abderhalden-Kaufmann-Lignac syndrome (cystinosis) E72.04 **Abdomen, abdominal** - see also condition
- acute R10.0
- angina K55.1
- muscle deficiency syndrome Q79.4
Abdominalgia - see Pain, abdominal
Abduction contracture, hip or other joint - see Contraction, joint

Table of Drugs ICD-9-CM

ICD-9 Table of Drugs and Biologicals

Substance	Poisoning	Accident	Therapeutic Use	Suicide Attempt	Assault	Undetermined
1-propanol	980.3	E860.4	-	E950.9	E962.1	E980.9
2-propanol	980.2	E860.3	-	E950.9	E962.1	E980.9
2, 4-D (dichlorophen-oxyacetic acid)	989.4	E863.5	-	E950.6	E962.1	E980.7
2, 4-toluene diisocyanate	983.0	E864.0	-	E950.7	E962.1	E980.6
2, 4, 5-T (trichloro-phenoxyacetic acid)	989.2	E863.5	-	E950.6	E962.1	E980.7
14-hydroxydihydro-morphinone	965.09	E850.2	E935.2	E950.0	E962.0	E980.0
ABOB	961.7	E857	E931.7	E950.4	E962.0	E980.4
Abrus (seed)	988.2	E865.3	-	E950.9	E962.1	E980.9
Absinthe	980.0	E860.1	-	E950.9	E962.1	E980.9

Table of Drugs ICD-10-CM

ICD-10 Table of Drugs and Biologicals

Substance	Poisoning Accidental Unintentional	Poisoning Intentional Self harm	Poisoning Assault	Poisoning undetermined	Adverse effect	Underdosing
1-propanol	T51.3x1	T51.3x2	T51.3x3	T51.3x4	—	—
2-propanol	T51.2x1	T51.2x2	T51.2x3	T51.2x4	—	—
2,4-D (dichlorophen-oxyacetic acid)	T60.3x1	T60.3x2	T60.3x3	T60.3x4	—	—
2,4-toluene diisocyanate	T65.0x1	T65.0x2	T65.0x3	T65.0x4	—	—
2,4,5-T (trichloro-phenoxyacetic acid)	T60.1x1	T60.1x2	T60.1x3	T60.1x4	—	—
14-hydroxydihydro-morphinone	T40.2x1	T40.2x2	T40.2x3	T40.2x4	T40.2x5	T40.2x6
ABOB	T37.5x1	T37.5x2	T37.5x3	T37.5x4	T37.5x5	T37.5x6
Abrine	T62.2x1	T62.2x2	T62.2x3	T62.2x4	—	—
Abrus (seed)	T62.2x1	T62.2x2	T62.2x3	T62.2x4	—	—
Absinthe	T51.0x1	T51.0x2	T51.0x3	T51.0x4	—	—
- beverage	T51.0x1	T51.0x2	T51.0x3	T51.0x4	—	—

Under ICD-9, Accidental poisoning by Absinthe would be 980.0.
Under ICD-10, this code would be T51.0x1
When looking at T51.0, you find this:
T51.0 Toxic effect of ethanol
Toxic effect of ethyl alcohol Excludes2: acute alcohol intoxication or "hangover" effects drunkenness pathological alcohol intoxication
T51.0x Toxic effect of ethanol
T51.0x1 Toxic effect of ethanol, accidental (unintentional)
Toxic effect of ethanol NOS

As a coder, we must understand that the disease doesn't change. Chicken Pox is still Chicken Pox, Measles is still Measles, and Chest Pain is still Chest Pain. The only thing that DOES change are the codes themselves.

Chicken Pox:

ICD-9-CM:

V05.4 Varicella
    Chicken pox

ICD-10-CM

B01.9 Varicella without complication

Measles

ICD-9-CM:

055 Measles
056 Rubella

ICD-10-CM

B05.9 - Measles without complication **B06.9** - Rubella without complication

Chest pain ICD-9-CM:

786.50 Chest pain, unspecified

ICD-10-CM

R07.9 - Chest pain, unspecified

Again, with ICD-9-CM, you have 3, 4, or 5 digit codes. With ICD-10-CM, you can have up to 7 digits with a code. That is one big difference between ICD-9-CM and ICD-10-CM.

Some guidelines exist in ICD-9-CM, but do not exist in ICD-10-CM. For example:

Some guidelines changed or do not exist in ICD-10

ICD-9
- 15. Admissions/Encounters for Rehabilitation
- When the purpose for the admission/encounter is rehabilitation, sequence the appropriate V code from category V57, Care involving use of rehabilitation procedures, as the principal/first-listed diagnosis. The code for the condition for which the service is being performed should be reported as an additional diagnosis.
- Only one code from category V57 is required. Code V57.89, Other specified rehabilitation procedures, should be assigned if more than one type of rehabilitation is performed during a single encounter. A procedure code should be reported to identify each type of rehabilitation therapy actually performed.

ICD-10
Does not exist in ICD-10

If you look at the following, you can see the differences between ICD-9-CM and ICD-10-CM

Chapter	ICD-9-CM	Descriptor	ICD-10-CM	Descriptor	# Codes **
1	001-139	Infectious and Parasitic Diseases	A00-B99	Certain infectious and parasitic diseases	455
2	140-239	Neoplasms	C00-D48	Neoplasms	622
3	240-279	Endocrine, Nutritional, and Metabolic Diseases and Immunity Disorders	D50-D89	Diseases of the blood and blood-forming organs and certain disorders involving the immune mechanism	696
4	280-289	Diseases of Blood and Blood Forming Organs	E00-E90	Endocrine, nutritional and metabolic diseases	2,230
5	290-319	Mental Disorders	F00-F99	Mental and behavioural disorders	1,163
6	320-389	Diseases of Nervous System and Sense Organs	G00-G99	Diseases of the nervous system	792
7	390-459	Diseases of Circulatory System	H00-H59	Diseases of the eye and adnexa	296
8	460-519	Diseases of Respiratory System	H60-H95	Diseases of the ear and mastoid process	214
9	520-579	Diseases of Digestive System	I00-I99	Diseases of the circulatory system	3,885
10	580-629	Diseases of Genitourinary System	J00-J99	Diseases of the respiratory system	1,439
11	630-677	Complications of Pregnancy, Childbirth, and the Puerperium	K00-K93	Diseases of the digestive system	1,560
12	680-709	Diseases Skin and Subcutaneous Tissue	L00-L99	Diseases of the skin and subcutaneous tissue	322
13	710-739	Diseases of Musculoskeletal and Connective Tissue	M00-M99	Diseases of the musculoskeletal system and connective tissue	1,374
14	740-759	Congenital Anomalies	N00-N99	Diseases of the genitourinary system	1,046
15	760-779	Newborn (Perinatal) Guidelines	O00-O99	Pregnancy, childbirth and the puerperium	600
16	780-799	Signs, Symptoms and Ill-Defined Conditions	P00-P96	Certain conditions originating in the perinatal period	213
17	800-999	Injury and Poisoning	Q00-Q99	Congenital malformations, deformations and chromosomal abnormalities	240
18	V01-V89	Classification of Factors Influencing Health Status and Contact with Health Service	R00-R99	Symptoms, signs and abnormal clinical and laboratory findings, not elsewhere classified	1,585
19	E800-E999	Supplemental Classification of External Causes of Injury and Poisoning	S00-T98	Injury, poisoning and certain other consequences of external causes	1,235
20			V01-98	External causes of morbidity and mortality	714
21			Z00-Z98	Factors influencing health status and contact with health services	2,441
22			U00-U99	Codes for special purposes	
				Total Codes	23,122

Note: ** Information Obtained from data compiled by AHA & AHIMA

Under ICD-9, you have 19 Chapters and under ICD-10, you have 22 Chapters.

ICD-9-CM codes are made up of 3, 4, or 5 numbers.

ICD-10-CM Codes are made up of a letter and numbers. ICD-10-CM codes can go as high as 7 digits.

Former V Codes are now Z Codes

- One of the most popular V Codes was the Well baby Check which used V20.2 Routine infant or child health check.

- Under ICD-10, this has been changed to
- Z00.1 Encounter for routine child health examination Encounter for development testing of infant or child Excludes1: health supervision of foundling or other healthy infant or child (Z76.1-Z76.2)
- Z00.10 Encounter for routine child health examination without abnormal findings Encounter for routine child health examination NOS
- Z00.11 Encounter for routine child health examination with abnormal findings
- Use additional code to identify abnormal findings

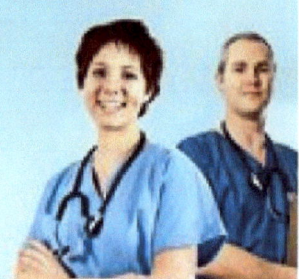

ICD-9-CM

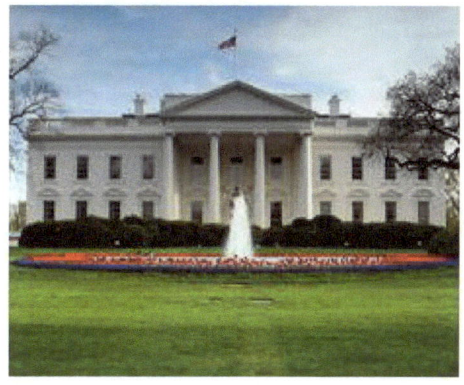

1600 Pennsylvania Avenue

ICD-10-CM

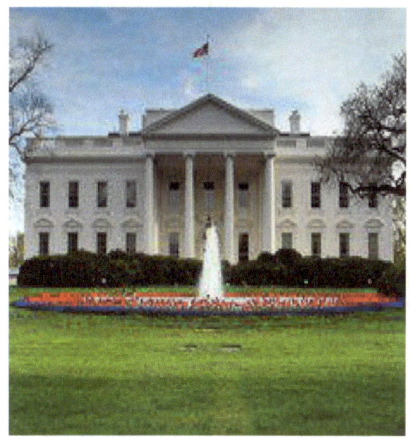

W01.9 Pennsylvania Avenue

What to do to be ready by October 1, 2013?

One thing you do not want to do is wait! You have much to do between now and when ICD-10 is effective on October 1, 2013.

1. YOU NEED TO BE READY FOR ANSI 5010

ANSI 5010 is the HIPAA approved code set for ICD-10. CMS has published a timeline to get ready for ICD-10-CM. This can be found here:

https://www.cms.gov/ICD_10/03_ICD-10andVersion5010ComplianceTimelines.asp#TopOfPage

Date	Compliance Step
January 1, 2010	Payers and providers should begin internal testing of Version 5010 standards for electronic claims
December 31, 2010	Internal testing of Version 5010 must be complete to achieve Level I Version 5010 compliance
January 1, 2011	• Payers and providers should begin external testing of Version 5010 for electronic claims • CMS begins accepting Version 5010 claims • Version 4010 claims continue to be
December 31, 2011	External testing of Version 5010 for electronic claims must be complete to achieve Level II Version 5010 compliance
January 1, 2012	• All electronic claims must use Version 5010 • Version 4010 claims are no longer accepted
October 1, 2013	• Claims for services provided on or after this date must use ICD-10 codes for medical diagnosis and inpatient procedures • CPT codes will continue to be used for outpatient services

2. You need to contact your medical coding/medical billing software vendors and clearinghouses to find out when they will make the necessary program changes and when they will start testing ANSI 5010 to be ready by the various timelines established by CMS and the various insurance companies. Your software will need to be able to handle both ICD-9-CM and ICD-10-CM. Why? On September 30, 2013, ICD-9 will still be effective. Although you may have a patient seen in 9/30/13, their visit will still be coded using ICD-9-CM. You may

have a patient that withheld insurance information until January 2014 or you may get an attorney or insurance company request for a claim for a date of service that is prior to October 1, 2013, so your software needs to keep the ICD-9-CM codes for these contingencies.

3. You need to make the appropriate changes to your practice or company coding policies and compliance plans.

4. Training and Certification

Your doctors, coders and billers need to be updated on ICD-10. Doctors must understand the importance of better documentation of a patient visit. This is because some ICD-10 codes are based on anatomical location. Poor or insufficient documentation could delay the claims process, which in turn, could result in a decline of practice revenue. Your coders may have to undergo retesting and recertification. That will be according to the certifying agency/organization/association. According to Rhonda Buckholtz of the AAPC: "*You will be required to complete an online competency exam on ICD-10-CM once the ruling becomes final. Your certification will be tied to it. We will more than likely give a grace period of 1 year before and a few months after for you to complete it. It will only include ICD-10-CM questions.*" If you have a person in your coding department, ensure that they undergo the proper coding training and, if required, certification. If you outsource, find out what they are doing to get their coders and company ready for ICD-10-CM. It could be very costly to find your claims denied, returned or pended due to coding errors. In-house training of your staff can be provided through recognized, accepted and reputable coding training and certifying organizations/agencies/companies. Be cautious of the fly-by-night companies that will pop up as we get closer to the effective date. Do not take credence with scare tactics some may try to present.

5. Update your superbills if they have any diagnosis codes on them. Remember, CPT will still be here. It is only ICD-9 that is making the huge change. CPT 93042 may still be here but 786.50 may not be the code to support it. Code R07.9 may be the code you use to support an EKG interpretation and report.

6. Ensure your coders and billers have current ICD-10-CM manuals. I recommend keeping your 2012-2013 ICD-9-CM manual for possible referencing, as the situation requires it.

7. If you are contracted with an insurance company and your contract demands compliance with the insurance company's coding policies, get with that insurance company to review the changes they are making, if any. Make sure that they meet industry standard guidelines and requirements.

8. If you need help, contact one of the coding/billing organizations/associations for assistance. Examples are the MAB, AAPC, PAHCS, POMAA, AHIMA, or State Hospital Association/Medical Societies.

9. Practice the Boy Scout Motto: "Be Prepared!"

10.   Never assume anything! VERIFY! VERIFY! VERIFY!

About the Author:

Goal-oriented medical professional with 15 years of combined civilian and military experience driven by a desire to provide top-notch Allied Health Education, experienced and skilled in curriculum writing, competency based education, and facilitative presentation of the Allied Health subject theorem and practicum. My approach, regarding subject conveyance, has consistently achieved significant results in the increasing allied health field.

References and Websites (Listed in no particular order):

Medical Association of Billers:
www.e-medbill.com and http://medicalassociationofbillers.yuku.com/

Professional Association of Healthcare Coding Specialists
www.pahcs.org

American Academy of Professional Coders
www.aapc.com

Physician Office Managers Association of America
www.pomaa.com

Billing-Coding Advantage (BC Advantage)
www.billing-coding.com

Don Self
www.donself.com

American Health Information Management Association
www.ahima.org

Centers for Medicare and Medicaid Services ICD-10
https://www.cms.gov/ICD10/

World Health Organization ICD-10
http://apps.who.int/classifications/apps/icd/icd10online/

Billing-Coding. Net
http://www.medicalbillingandcoding.net/medical_billers_forum.htm

American Medical Association ICD-10 http://www.ama-assn.org/ama/pub/physician-resources/solutions-managing-your-practice/codingbilling-insurance/hipaahealth-insurance-portability-accountability-act/transaction-code-setstandards/icd10-code-set.shtml

National Uniform Claim Commission
http://www.nucc.org/

www.ingramcontent.com/pod-product-compliance
Lightning Source LLC
Chambersburg PA
CBHW041307180526
45172CB00003B/1010